The Layman's Guide to Medical School

Viruses

CONTENTS

INTRODUCTION

There's one thing every person in the entire world has, and it's a body. Maybe that will change in the future, but for now, I can guarantee that if you're reading this book, you have a body. The good and bad thing about the body is that it's incredibly complex, both by itself and in the way it interacts with the outside world. Before I started medical school, I knew that the body was complicated and that things affected it, but not how. When I started school, I realized that, while there are countless ways in which the body can change based on its interaction with the world, the complexity lies there, not in the individual details. I decided then and there that there's no reason people shouldn't learn about how their body works—without needing to pay a few hundred thousand dollars for the privilege. After all, taking care of your body is the best way you can ensure you lead a healthy, and therefore happy, life.

I started *The Layman's Guide to Medical School* to bring the information I learn in medical school to everyone. I won't use big Latin words (too often) or write in the convoluted way that bores the heck out of you. I'll just explain, as concisely as I can, what the body does, why it does it, and why we care. I also have often found that non-fiction books have 50 pages of good material and 150 of filler, so I've decided to cut out the filler and keep only the interesting parts.

If you have questions about the books, requests for new topics, or general feedback, you can email me at laymansmedicalschool@gmail.com. You can also sign up for the mailing list there; just send me an email with "Mailing List" as the subject.

One disclaimer: I am not (yet) a doctor, and this book is not intended to diagnose you or recommend treatment. For that, you need to see a real doctor.

Thanks for downloading the book, and happy reading!

Colleen Fleshman

30 December 2014

VIRAL OVERVIEW

To understand viruses, we need to understand a little bit about the human body. Our body is composed of trillions of cells, which is, frankly, such a high number it's impossible to understand. Since each one of us doesn't take up the entire Earth, we can conclude that cells are very small. In fact, a cell can't be seen with the naked eye. Microscopes allow us to peer into cells, and between that and a large group of scientists willing to spend decades performing experiment after experiment, we have a pretty good idea of what goes on inside the human cell.

So what *is* going on inside that cell? There are a lot of things going on in there, so much so that hundreds of books have been written on the topic. For our purposes, we just need to know a little about RNA and DNA. If you're already familiar with the concepts, you can skip the next three paragraphs.

DNA is short for deoxyribonucleic acid, but since that's too much of a mouthful, we'll stick with DNA. RNA is ribonucleic acid, which is a little easier to say but not much, so we'll go with RNA as well. DNA is the basic building block of life. You can think of it as a blueprint for our bodies. DNA tells the manufacturing system of the cell what proteins to make, and these proteins are what handle a lot of the fun functions of our body.

Every single cell in our body has the same copy of DNA. In biology, there's something called the central dogma, which is this: DNA → RNA → protein. In other words, DNA gets transcribed into RNA, which gets translated into protein. The basic blueprint, DNA, contains too much information to tackle at once, so memos get sent out in the form of RNA that encode for one protein. That protein is then assembled using the protein-making machine, also known as a ribosome (which is also a protein). Then the proteins run off and do their stuff, which we won't get into here. Suffice it to say, without DNA we'd be nothing.

Let's look a little closer at DNA, because understanding DNA is key to understanding how viruses work. To make DNA, we take a set of four nucleic acids, which is a sugar bound to a phosphate and one of four bases, and combine them in various ways. Think of a set of blocks where you have countless blocks in only four colors: green, red, blue, and yellow. Although you only have four colors to choose from, you can combine them in any number of unique ways to make up unique segments of DNA called genes. For instance, you can take 5 red (R), 4 yellow (Y), 3 blue (B), and 1 green (G) to make: RRYGBRYYBRBRY, RYBRRRGYBYYRB, and countless other combinations. When you consider that you can change the number of each one of the four blocks, you start to realize that there are limitless ways you can arrange the DNA. Each of these combinations codes for a unique protein, so you can imagine that we can make a lot of proteins that do a lot of things in the body.

In order to make those proteins, we send out bits of RNA

to get translated into proteins. The RNA pieces are exact copies of the DNA, but instead of copying the entire DNA strand, we only copy a small part, such as RRYGBRYYBRBRY (note that these letters are based on colors, not the real RNA and DNA letters. For more details on that, check out *The Layman's Guide to Medical School: The Cell*). These small bits of RNA go out and get made into proteins by ribosomes, as we mentioned earlier.

What does this have to do with viruses? You ask. Don't worry, we're getting to that. Now that we understand a little about DNA, we can talk about viruses. Viruses are fascinating because, unlike bacteria, fungi, lions, and other things that can hurt us, viruses are not alive. I'll let that sink in for a minute. Remember that cold you had last winter, when you felt like your head was so clogged you couldn't hold it up? That was caused by something that ISN'T EVEN ALIVE. If the virus were getting some sort of life support out of my body, like bacteria do, I would understand why it needs to infect me. Not viruses. They're basically mindless drones sent out to attack without any real purpose. It's annoying.

Viruses aren't dead, either. We should get that straight. Viruses are more like a saucepan. Saucepans aren't alive, but I wouldn't call them dead. They just exist. Now, because viruses aren't alive, they're pretty basic and they're pretty small. Viruses are made up of only a few things: DNA or RNA, a capsid made of proteins, and sometimes, an envelope. We'll explain what these are in a minute. First, let's talk about the nucleic acids, which are DNA and RNA.

Viral DNA and RNA are the same as human DNA and

RNA. The same, except that the order of those nucleic acids is different, so they code for different proteins that do different things than our proteins. The important distinction to know is that viruses, unlike human cells, can use RNA as their basic blueprint instead of DNA. This becomes critically important, as we'll discuss in the section on Infection. What we need to know right now is that the virus can either have DNA or RNA, and that genetic material can either be one long strand, one circular strand, or a bunch of strands.

Viral capsids are a protective outer layer of proteins that also happens to give viruses a lot of their pathogenicity (pathogenicity is a fancy term for "how this thing makes us sick"). Every virus has a capsid, and it comes in only one of two shapes: helical or icosahedral. Helical capsids look like a very twisty waterslide, and icosahedral capsids look like a 60-sided gem. For our purposes, that's really all we need to know about capsids right now.

Envelopes are only found on some viruses, and they make a huge difference in how the virus can spread. An envelope is composed of a membrane of lipids (fats) and proteins, and they're similar to the membranes that are found on all human cells. If a virus has an envelope, it's called an enveloped virus. If it doesn't have an envelope, it's called a naked capsid virus, or naked virus for short. It's unfortunate for us that more viruses aren't worried about their modesty, because enveloped viruses are a lot less stable than naked viruses. That's because the envelope of a virus must stay wet, and it can be destroyed by heat and acid (like the acid found in the stomach). Naked capsid viruses don't need to worry about that, so they can live on surfaces like doorknobs and kitchen tables without worrying about drying out or getting killed by that vinegar you rubbed on the tabletop. They also can survive your stomach, which is highly acidic (as anyone who's had acid reflux knows), so they can infect you even if you swallow them. When we look at individual viruses, we'll talk about how they spread and where they can infect you, and the envelope is the major deciding factor in that discussion.

So that's a virus, and that's all that a virus is. It doesn't have machinery for making energy, so it can't replicate or do anything that requires energy on its own. And that, my friend, is why viruses infect humans. They steal our energy and replication machinery (more on this in the Infection section) and make copies of themselves. Despite not being alive, viruses have a strong desire to make more of themselves, and therefore we get sick.

CLASSIFICATION OF VIRUSES

Now that we've covered the basics of viruses, let's talk classification. I can hear those of you who took biology groaning right now.

"Classification," you're saying, "is boring and pointless."

Honestly, some if it is. Sometimes I think biologists classify for classification's sake, but in the case of viruses, there's a purpose. Classification of viruses can tell us something about the mechanism they use to infect human cells, which is very important when it comes to trying to stop them. I promise to make this classification as painless as possible, and if you really can't stand it, skip to the next chapter.

When it comes to classification, we start with the very basics: does the virus use DNA or RNA for its genetic code? If it uses DNA, we call it a DNA virus. Can you guess what we call RNA viruses? Darn, I gave the answer away. So far, we have:

| DNA | | RNA |

So far, so good. The next way we classify viruses is by the shape of the capsid, which we discussed earlier. The shape isn't critical to our discussion, so we'll just show the classification and move on.

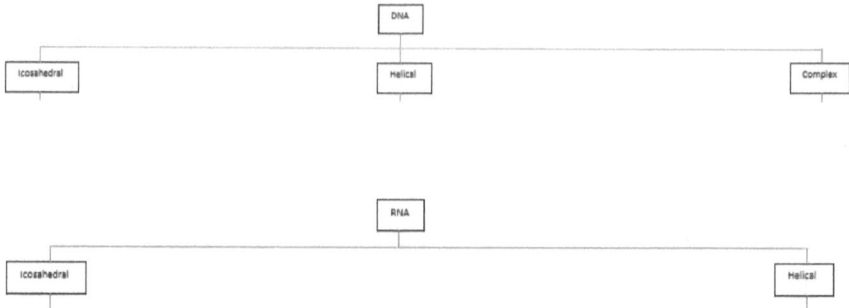

After the capsid shape, we classify the viruses by whether they're enveloped or naked. If you recall from the Overview section (which you should, it wasn't very long ago), enveloped viruses have an envelope that makes them susceptible to drying out. Naked viruses don't have that envelope and can therefore survive for long periods of time on surfaces outside the human (or other animal) body.

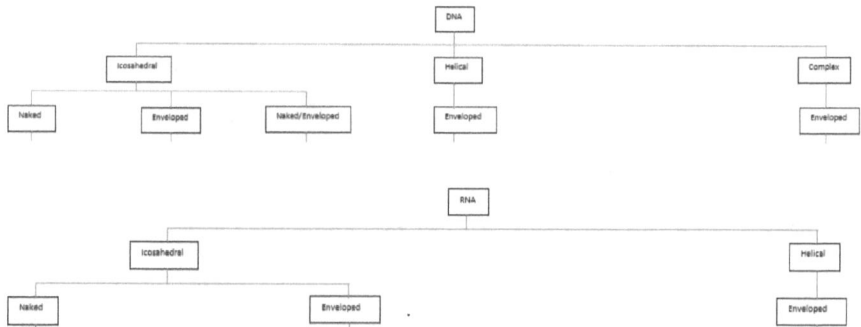

Next, we classify viruses by the shape of their nucleic acid (remember, nucleic acids are DNA and RNA), which can be linear, circular, or segmented. We also specify here if the RNA is positive sense or negative sense (more on this in the Infection section). I know this sounds really boring, but it becomes important later. When we get to the section on the flu, this will all make sense, I promise.

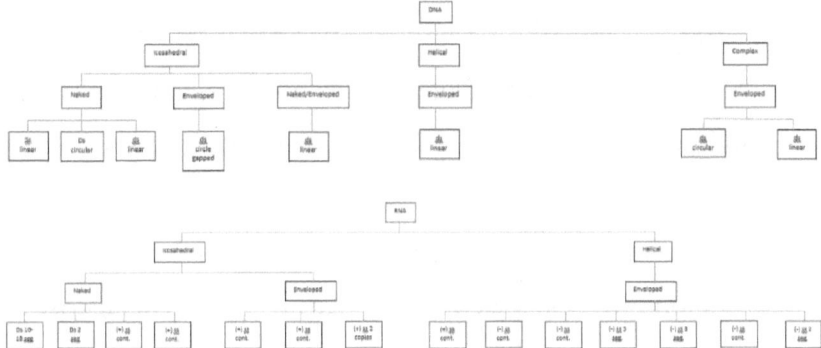

Great, are we done yet? Almost! Hang in there! There are a few more things that are used to classify viruses, but we're only going to look at the last relevant part, which is the viral families. This part is fairly simple because the families line up perfectly with the categories we already have. The family names can refer to a characteristic of the virus, like the retroviruses that go "retro" (back) from RNA to DNA, but they don't necessarily all follow that rule. For now, we'll put the list up to be complete, and as we talk about each disease, we'll refer back to this chart so you can understand how viruses are grouped.

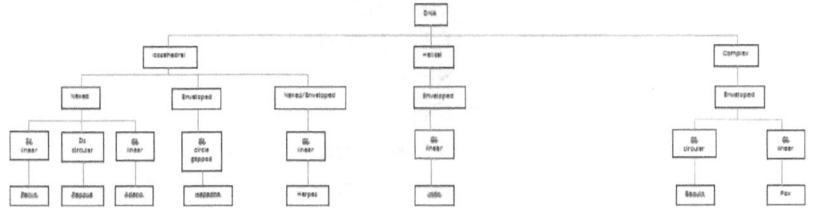

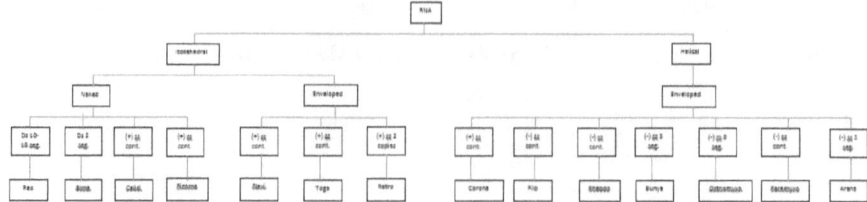

The interesting part of all of this is not so much how the viruses are categorized, but what diseases they actually cause and why these classifications affect the way they infect. We'll talk about infection in the next section, but for your reference, here's a chart of the common diseases caused by the virus families. The diseases in bold are the ones we'll discuss in this book. This is not a comprehensive list because that would be extensive, but it should give you an idea of what diseases are caused by these viruses.

	Family	Diseases
DNA	Parvoviridae	5th childhood exanthema (B19)
	Papovaviridae	Progressive Multifocal Encephalopathy (JC virus) Nephropathy (BK virus) Genital warts (Human Papilloma Virus (HPV))
	Adenoviridae	Upper respiratory tract infection
	Hepadnaviridae	Hepatitis
	Herpesviridae	**Cold Sores (HSV-1)** **Genital warts (HSV-2)** **Chickenpox (VZV)** **Shingles (VZV)** Cytomegalovirus (CMV) **Mononucleosis (EBV)** Kaposi sarcoma (HHV-8)
	Poxviridae	Smallpox Skin warts (Molluscum contagiosum)

RNA	Reoviridae	**Rotavirus** **Colorado Tick Fever (Coltivirus)**
	Caliciviridae	Norovirus
	Picornaviridae	**Common Cold (Rhinovirus)** Polio (Poliovirus) Coxsackie (Coxsackie virus) Hepatitis A
	Flaviviridae	**Yellow Fever** **Dengue** West Nile Hepatitis C
	Togaviridae	**Rubella**
	Retroviridae	CTLV **HIV**
	Coronaviridae	**Common Cold** **SARS**
	Filoviridae	Marburg **Ebola**
	Rhabdoviridae	Rabies
	Bunyaviridae	**Korean Hemorrhagic Fever and Renal Syndrome (Hantavirus)** **Hantavirus Pulmonary Syndrome (Sin Nombre virus)**
	Orthomyxoviridae	**Influenza**
	Paramyxoviridae	**Measles (Morbillivirus)** **Mumps (Mumps virus)** Parainfluenza Respiratory Syncyntial Virus
	Arenaviridae	Lassa Fever (Lassa Fever virus)

INFECTION

Now that we've gotten our viruses neatly organized, let's talk about infection. This is the fun part anyway. In this chapter, we'll talk about how viruses infect our body and what happens when they do.

As I mentioned in the overview section, viruses can't replicate on their own. They're so small they can't fit a whole lot of DNA or RNA into their capsid, so they have to make do with only the bare necessities. Poxvirus, which is the largest virus family, has only, at most, 280 kilobases, which is a fancy way of saying 280,000 base pairs. In contrast, the human genome probably has 3.2 billion base pairs. So as you can see, viruses don't have a lot of extra DNA/RNA space to encode for proteins to make copies of themselves. What they do instead is hijack our cells' machinery to replicate. Because of this, viruses are known as obligate intracellular pathogens, which just means they can't replicate without being inside of a cell. This doesn't mean they can't exist outside the cell, because if that were true, they would never get transmitted between people.

To understand the infection and transmission path of a virus, let's follow one virus on its journey. We'll look at a rhinovirus, which is one of the causes of the common cold. The rhinovirus is a naked capsid virus, so it can survive on fomites, which means any surface, such as tables, doorknobs, etc. So let's say someone with a cold sneezed onto her hand and grabbed a doorknob. A few minutes later, you walk up and grab that same doorknob. The rhinovirus gets transferred onto your hand. When your nose itches a moment later, you raise your hand and rub it across your nostrils. Just like that, the virus is inside you. The nose is actually the rhinovirus's favorite location because it's a slightly lower temperature than the rest of your body, and the rhinovirus prefers temperatures lower than 33 Celsius (the human body is 37 Celsius).

Now that the virus is inside your body, it needs to get inside a cell. This first step in doing this is called attachment, and it's occurs when a receptor on the virus latches onto a receptor on your cell. This step determines what cells a virus can infect because receptors on cells vary based on the type of cell. In the human body, receptors are used for a wide variety of things, including getting nutrients like glucose into the cell, responding to stimuli by nerves, and a whole host of interactions with the environment outside the cell. Because each type of cell has different functions and different needs, the receptors vary. The receptor on the virus is configured to attach to certain receptors on human cells, so the virus is restricted in which cells it can infect based on whether or not they express the receptor the virus can recognize. Most of the strains of the rhinovirus recognize a receptor called ICAM-1, which is found on a lot of cells, so it can infect a wide variety of cells. The receptor is also a good target for antiviral drugs, since if you can prevent the virus from getting into the cell, you can stop its replication.

Once the virus has attached to the cell, it needs to get through the membrane, a step called penetration. Get your mind out of the gutter; it's not that kind of penetration. This is just the movement of the virus into the cell, and it's often coupled with a step called uncoating, where the virus loses its envelope (if present) and its capsid. Uncoating needs to occur in order for the viral DNA or RNA to be used to make copies, and it can occur at the same time as penetration, or directly after.

The method for actually getting into the cell varies based on the type of virus. The really small viruses, like picorna, can fit in between the lipid bilayer of the cell membrane (for details on the cell, see *The Layman's Guide to Medical School: The Cell*) and directly infect the cell. Rhinovirus—the cold-causing virus, if you've forgotten—is in the picornaviridae family, so this is how it gets inside the cell. Most of the larger viruses aren't able to do this, though. These ones have two ways of getting inside: fusion and endocytosis.

Fusion occurs when the virus attaches to the cell and the envelope of the virus fuses with the cell membrane. This method is primarily used by enveloped viruses, as it allows them to send in the naked capsid while the envelope just becomes a part of the cell membrane.

Endocytosis occurs when the cell engulfs the virus in its membrane. Think of a water droplet rolling over a crumb. The crumb ends up inside the water droplet, but it's still a separate entity. With the cell, the virus hits the membrane and the membrane folds around it like a pocket of dough around the meat of a calzone. The endosome (calzone, in our analogy) is taken into the cell, where the virus can trick the cell into uncoating it. Let's take a look at uncoating next.

Uncoating can also occur via a few different processes, depending on the structure of the virus. For some, binding to the receptor on the cell's surface can cause the virus to change shape, so that the contents of the virus—meaning the DNA or RNA—can be released into the cell without its capsid. For those in endosomes (the calzone, remember?), the preferred method is acid. Not the drug, just acid itself, which is a high load of protons. A lot of viruses carry a protein with them that pumps protons into the endosome, creating a high-acid environment that breaks down the capsid on the viral DNA or RNA and sets it free.

Now that the virus is free, it's actually no longer able to infect cells. Viruses need the capsid, with its proteins, in order to infect a cell. However, it can't replicate without taking the capsid off. So why do we care? Well, if we can stop the viruses after they uncoat but before they replicate, we can prevent the virus from infecting any other cell. Some antivirals take advantage of this. We'll talk more about antivirals later.

The next step is the most important one in the overall infectivity: replication. The reason this is so important is that when you get infected with a virus, you usually get infected with only a small number of viruses. If that number doesn't increase, your body will pretty easily be able to kill off the few that infected you.

In order to cause a noticeable infection, the viruses have to replicate and build up a high viral load, which just means that there are a lot of viruses. Once the viral load gets high enough, you begin to show symptoms of whatever illness is infecting you, and you're also contagious to other people. But how does replication actually occur?

As we discussed in the overview section, viruses and contain either RNA or DNA as their basic blueprint. DNA viruses have it a little easier when it comes to replication. As I mentioned earlier, humans have DNA, and we need to be able to replicate that DNA in order to make new cells of our own. Therefore, DNA viruses simply hijack our DNA replication machinery and put it to use for themselves. It's simple, elegant, and unfortunately, highly effective. As you can probably imagine, using our own body against us makes it easy for the viruses to hide. Our immune system has ways around this (you can learn more in *The Layman's Guide to Medical School: The Immune System*), but you'll see when we discuss herpes that viruses are very good at hiding from our immune system. That means they're also annoyingly good at hiding from drugs that target them, and the only way to get rid of viruses is to kill the cell they're infecting. The upshot of this is that a lot of the symptoms you show when you get infected with a virus, such as a fever, muscle aches, and that annoying runny nose are not caused by the virus itself, but by your body trying to get rid of it.

That's DNA viruses in a nutshell, but what about RNA viruses? I mentioned before that in the human cell, we always go from DNA to RNA. RNA never gets copied from itself, and so we don't have anything that can make RNA from RNA. This means that all RNA viruses have to carry a protein with them that can do that replication for them. These proteins are termed polymerases, which is a general term for a protein that replicates DNA or RNA, and they can either be RNA-dependent RNA polymerases or RNA-dependent DNA polymerases. These sound a little wordy, but if you break down what they're actually saying, the "RNA-dependent" part refers to the fact that the polymerases need premade RNA to copy—they depend on the RNA already in the virus. In RNA-dependent RNA polymerases, RNA is made from RNA – the protein polymerizes (makes) RNA. In RNA-dependent DNA polymerases, DNA is made from RNA. Another term for viruses that carry RNA-dependent DNA polymerases is retroviruses, the most famous of which is HIV. The "retro-" refers to the fact that the virus goes backwards in the normal chain – from RNA to DNA instead of the other way around. Retroviruses then hijack our DNA replication machinery, just like DNA viruses. We'll discuss retroviruses more when we talk about HIV.

The other thing of note is that viruses don't carry any sort of proof-reading mechanism with them. You can imagine that when a copy of either DNA or RNA is getting made, it would be pretty easy to accidentally put in the wrong base at one of those millions of sites. Since we humans like our DNA to stay pretty much the same, we have a number of proof-reading mechanisms to ensure that mistakes get fixed. Viruses don't care. They want to grow at an unregulated pace, which in human cells leads to cancer. If they're DNA viruses and are using our machinery, we proofread the copies for them (it's not that we're nice; our cells are just built to always proofread). The advantage here is that DNA viruses are less likely to have a beneficial mutation that lets them circumvent some of our immune system's defenses. RNA viruses don't have any sort of proofreading, so they're constantly mutating as mistakes accumulate. We'll talk about this more in the influenza section.

While copies of the genetic material (DNA or RNA) are accumulating, the viruses also use our machinery to make proteins from their genetic material. These proteins can be used to attach to other cells, to release the genetic material once the virus is inside a cell, or they can be polymerases that help make more virus copies. Regardless, each virus needs a complete set of these proteins, just like the first virus that infected the cell had them. Only with all of these proteins can the new virus infect more cells.

Once the virus has made a bunch of copies of itself, it needs to get out of the cell so it can infect other cells. There are a couple methods, but the main difference you'll see is between the naked and enveloped viruses. The naked ones don't want anything covering them, so they need to break through the cell membrane to get out. This occurs via a process called lysis, which is a fancy way of saying it breaks open the cell membrane and escapes. Cells don't do well with holes in their membranes, so these cells pretty much all die.

For enveloped viruses, they need a membrane, and the membrane of the human cell is good enough for them. Many enveloped viruses will actually put the pieces of the virus together on the cell membrane surface and then pinch off a bit of the membrane in a process called budding. These cells survive to replicate and assemble more viruses, while the newly assembled viruses flit off to infect more cells.

That's the basic process of the infection cycle. It's amazingly elegant, and by using our own machinery against us, it allows viruses to stay small and have an even easier time hiding from our immune system. Just because they can hide doesn't mean we never find them, though. Next we'll discuss antivirals and vaccines that can protect us from these pesky viruses.

ANTIVIRALS

This is a very important thing to know: antibiotics do NOTHING against viruses. That means that when you have the flu and your doctor tells you to sleep it off, she's right. If your doctor tries to prescribe you antibiotics, just tell her "No thanks, the flu is caused by a virus and I don't want to promote antibiotic-resistant strains of bacteria." The added bonus here is you get to sound smarter than your doctor.

The reason antibiotics don't work is because they're designed to target bacteria, and they do so by specifically attacking parts of the bacteria, like their outer protein layer or their replication machinery, that are bacteria-specific. We do this because we don't want to kill off our own cells. The problem with viruses is that they use our own cells to replicate, so they're much harder to target. Until the eighties, people thought it was impossible to selectively target the virus without chemotherapy-like side effects of slaughtering our own cells. The good news is people were wrong. In 1982, a couple of scientists developed acyclovir, which selectively targets the herpes virus while leaving our cells (mostly) alone. Those scientists won a Nobel Prize. Since then, a number of antivirals have come to market that target various viruses.

"Antivirals?" You say. "Those sound great! Why doesn't my doctor give me those when I have the flu?"

For one thing, antivirals are only effective against certain viruses. Secondly, antivirals can be very expensive, and when you're a healthy individual, you're going to be able to fight off the flu using your own immune system. And finally, one effect of some antivirals is to cause flu-like symptoms. It's pretty pointless to prescribe something that's going to cause the same effect as the actual illness! Not every antiviral does this, of course, but there are some that cause issues, and it's probably not really going to help you fight the flu much faster.

These days, though, better and better antivirals are coming to the market with fewer side effects. You've probably even seen a few advertised on television such as oseltamivir, which you probably know better as Tamiflu®, and rimantidine (Flumadine®). The recommendations vary on whether or not these are actually beneficial in healthy individuals, with some groups saying they should be prescribed to most everyone and others saying the risks are too great, but the point is they exist. But how do they work?

If you were paying attention in the replication section, you may have noticed that all RNA viruses have to carry their own special protein to help them replicate. This makes an excellent target for antivirals because it's unique to the virus, so you don't have to worry about accidentally killing off our cells. This is far from the only target, though. Other targets include the uncoating step, which rimantidine targets, and the release from the cell, which is what aseltamivir targets. Anything that's unique to the virus can be a target. And this, my friends, is why knowing each tiny protein in every cell in the human body actually matters. Good work, research scientists.

DNA viruses are a little tougher to target because of their use of our machinery to replicate. Right now, drugs primarily focus on specific enzymes the viruses use to make their DNA preferentially replicated. This is the site that acyclovir targets.

In general, antivirals are great for the tougher viruses to fight and can be put to good use in immunocompromised people. They're not perfect, but they're a great step in the right direction.

VACCINES

Let's talk vaccines. I'm not here to preach about the good or evil of vaccines, or discuss if they cause autism. Well, maybe a few words on that. They don't. Vaccines don't cause autism and they aren't part of some government plot to weaken our children. That doesn't even make sense. The government has far more efficient ways to go after the people if it wanted to. One of the biggest things in medicine these days is a focus on evidence-based medicine, which is where we treat patients based on evidence gathered from scientific studies done using sound research methods. Studies have shown no link between autism and vaccines. I'm not saying that studies are infallible or that vaccines are perfect. All I'm saying is that as the intelligent person that you are, you should be aware of the difference between anecdotal evidence and scientifically-supported evidence.

I also don't necessarily think a vaccine is needed for everything. Some vaccines do contain adjuvants, which are essentially toxins intended to provoke a strong immune response so that you build a proper immunity to whatever you're being vaccinated against. This isn't a conspiracy; it's a necessary part of the vaccine in order to ensure that it works, and adjuvants are thoroughly tested before they're allowed into a vaccine. Some vaccines are also less effective than actually having the illness. If you're a young, healthy person who doesn't spend time with immunocompromised people (such as the elderly, young children, or people with HIV), I don't think you need a flu vaccine. The manufacturers often guess wrong on the strains that will be circulating anyway, making the vaccine ineffective. I'm probably annoying some pharmaceutical CEO, but I don't care. My point is that there's a time and a place for vaccines, and you, as a patient, should use your own sound judgment to decide if you want a particular vaccine.

The question, then, is when are vaccines useful? They're particularly effective against viruses that only have one serotype, which is just a fancy word for strain. We're all familiar with the different strains of the flu, since every ten years or so a new strain pops up and we name it things like H1N1 (more on that in the flu section). Some viruses have many strains, while others only have a handful or just one. Vaccines are particularly useful against viruses that have only one strain, so that your body can create an immune response to the vaccine and then recognize the virus as the same thing when it attempts to infect you.

Vaccines are also more useful against serious illnesses. Even if it were possible to create a vaccine against the common cold (we'll discuss this in the section on colds), it probably wouldn't be worth it because the worst the cold will do to you is make your nose run a bit. I don't think it would stop people from lining up down the street to get a vaccine if it were available, and I'd be right in that line with you, but it's not necessary for our long-term well-being.

Finally, vaccines are useful against common illnesses. If five people in the entire world have been infected with a virus and that number isn't growing, the pharmaceutical companies probably won't waste time and money developing a vaccine. That's just the reality of the medical industry. This isn't to say that vaccines aren't developed against rare illnesses. They certainly are. It's just to say that it's not likely, and it's even less likely that ordinary people like you and I will receive this vaccine.

Interesting fact about vaccines: the word "vaccine" is derived from the Latin *vaca*, which means "cow." This is a reference to the first vaccine, which was developed by Edward Jenner against smallpox. The vaccine was made from the cowpox virus, hence the name.

At this point, you're probably wondering how vaccines actually work. Vaccines work by tricking your immune system into thinking your body is getting infected by a disease without actually infecting your body. Think of the chickenpox. When we were kids, we all were rubbed against each other and forced to get chickenpox at a young age so that our body would build an immunity to it. My mom actually chucked me in the bathtub with my brother when he was sick until I ended up covered in red spots too. My immune system fought off the chickenpox virus eventually, and as a part of that response, it created cells known as memory cells that can recognize the chickenpox virus, should it ever infect me again. Because my body is primed for this particular virus, if it does get inside me, my body will kill it off before the viral load gets too high and I start showing symptoms. Pretty cool system, huh?

A vaccine works in the same way. There are a few different versions of vaccines: those that are inactivated, or dead bits of virus, and those that are live attenuated, which means that the actual virus in the vaccine is alive but has been modified so that it can't really infect you. Live attenuated vaccines become a problem for immunocompromised people, but for the rest of us, they're great.

Inactivated viruses are composed of proteins and other components of viruses or bacteria that are taken from the actual pathogen (virus or bacteria) after it has been killed. The proteins allow your immune cells to recognize a part of the pathogen and get activated, so that the next time the actual virus or bacteria shows up, those same cells will recognize it and wipe it out. The problem with inactivated vaccines is that they're not very immunogenic on their own, which means the body doesn't always recognize the need to mount a big immune response to dead cells. Our body is unfortunately clever that way. This is where adjuvants come in. Alum is the adjuvant used in vaccines, and it triggers a stronger response because alum is a toxin. It won't kill you, but your body certainly doesn't like it, so it mounts a response that allows the memory cells we talked about earlier to be activated. The injected polio vaccine is an example of an inactivated vaccine.

Live attenuated vaccines are the other form of vaccine commonly used. These are pathogens that are actually alive but have been modified so they aren't very infective. That way, our body responds properly because this is a real invasion, but the virus can't really infect us. Adjuvants aren't needed for live attenuated vaccines because our body recognizes them as an actual threat. The MMR vaccine is an example of a live attenuated vaccine.

Vaccines are one of the most revolutionary changes in medicine, since they allow us to completely avoid some really nasty illnesses. We should all thank Edward Jenner for that.

COLDS

The common cold is called common for a reason – it's very common. We all have had a cold (or two, or fifty) in our lifetimes. Now that you know a little about viruses, you might start wondering why we get so many colds, while other viruses are rare. There are a few reasons for this. The first is that there are over a hundred serotypes of the viruses that cause the cold. A serotype is a different version of the same virus, like when people talk about flu strains. The virus itself is the same, but there are some small differences in the RNA of the virus that let it infect you over and over again. On top of the various strains, there are actually multiple viruses that can cause the cold. We'll discuss two in particular in this section: the rhinovirus and the coronavirus.

The second reason that you come down with so many colds is that your immunity to colds gradually dissipates. Without going into details on how the immune system works, since that would take forever, just know that your body has two targeted ways of dealing with viruses. The first is called cell-mediated immunity, and it's where your body uses a type of immune cell called T cells to target viruses inside of the cell. For whatever reason, this doesn't work very well on naked viruses, and rhinoviruses and coronaviruses are both naked capsid viruses. The second type of immune response is called humoral immunity (a reference to the fluids, or "humors," in your body), and it works by having another immune cell called a B cell release antibodies into your blood to target the viruses outside the cell. This works well, but if your body isn't re-infected with the same cold strain within about eighteen months, this so-called humoral immunity dissipates. This isn't to say that you don't still have some immunity, but if you get the same cold strain again, you'll still show some symptoms of the cold before your body can fight it off.

So that's the bad news about colds. The good news is that the viruses are self-limiting, meaning that the worst that happens with a cold is you have a runny nose and maybe ache a little bit. Let's talk a little about what happens when a cold virus infects you.

As I mentioned, there are two main culprits indicted in the cold, and the rhinovirus is the more common of the two. Most of the time you have a cold, you have one of the rhinovirus serotypes inside of you. Remember in the infection section when we talked about the viruses getting inside of your cells? As I mentioned then, the rhinovirus uses the ICAM receptor, which is found on most cells lining your body, to attach to the cell. It then slides inside because it's so small and can easily cross into the body. One thing of note is that the rhinovirus actually prefers temperatures below 33°C, which is about 4 degrees lower than the human core temperature (4 Celsius degrees, that is. It's about 8 degrees in Fahrenheit, for those of us who struggle with the C/F conversions). This is part of the reason the cold virus is self-limiting: it can't survive in most cells in the body and prefers the extremities that are colder. In particular, it prefers the nose.

Once inside, the rhinovirus needs to uncoat and start replicating. Rhinoviruses are RNA viruses, which, if you'll recall, means they need to bring their own RNA-dependent RNA polymerase with them to start the replication process. They happen to be positive-sense RNA viruses, so they can start making proteins right away before copies get made.

Your body isn't sitting idly by while this happens. As the virus starts replicating, the infected cells send out distress signals to call immune cells to themselves. These signals make the gaps between cells lining blood vessels bigger, so that the immune cells can leak out of the bloodstream and attack the virus. This recruitment of your own immune defenses leads to an accumulation of fluid in the area, and since we already know that the rhinovirus prefers your nose, you end up with a runny nose. One of the "fun" things about viruses is most of the symptoms they cause aren't actually directly caused by the virus but are a result of your body trying to kill off the virus. Sometimes our body isn't too clever.

Because there are so many strains of the rhinovirus, vaccines are ineffective. There aren't too many drugs that do much either, and for the most part, your best bet is to just wait it out. Most colds only last 7-10 days, and while those days won't be pleasant, it's not the end of the world. There are a few drugs developed to stop the rhinovirus, but they only shorten it by a few days and some have weird side effects, like losing your sense of smell. I'll stick with the cold, personally.

Now that we've discussed the rhinovirus, let's talk about the coronavirus. No, it's not a beer-loving virus. Coronaviruses are so named because the scientists who first saw them under a microscope thought they looked like little suns with a corona around them, so they called them coronaviruses.

The coronavirus causes between 10 and 35% of colds, and it typically strikes when the rhinovirus isn't as widespread. It, like the rhinovirus, is a positive-sense RNA virus, so it can instantly produce proteins and needs its own special polymerase to replicate its RNA. What's strange about coronavirus, though, is that it's an enveloped virus that can survive the GI tract. I know, I told you earlier that only the naked viruses survived the GI tract. Unfortunately, nothing in biology is 100% or it would be a lot easier to treat people. What this means is that, along with the usual cold symptoms you see with a rhinovirus, a cold caused by a coronavirus can also cause diarrhea. Just in case you weren't uncomfortable enough with the runny nose and stuffed-up head.

The really, truly interesting thing about the coronavirus is that a new strain of it was discovered in 2003. If you can think back to 2003 and remember what virus panic was sweeping the world, you'll correctly guess that the coronavirus causes Severe Acute Respiratory Syndrome, better known as SARS.

Before you start panicking, you should know that the SARS strain of the coronavirus is rare. The common, cold-causing strains are a lot more likely to infect you. The SARS strain lives in animals and is believed to have crossed to humans from an animal, possibly a civet. Of course, we can't be entirely sure, but I can tell you that you probably won't ever get infected with SARS. But like I said, nothing in biology is 100%.

SARS does cause cold-like symptoms because it infects the cells in the nose and causes them to send out the same distress signals that the rhinovirus does. However, SARS also has an interesting mechanism in the respiratory tract where it binds to an ACE receptor (ACE like ACE inhibitors for the heart. It's the same receptor) and gets into the bloodstream. Once it's in the bloodstream, it causes fever, tiredness, headache, myalgia (muscle aches), a cough, and trouble breathing. About a quarter of the people who have SARS also get diarrhea, so it's extra fun for them.

For the most part, if you have a cold, you have a rhinovirus inside of the cells in your nose. You'll likely get a runny nose and a congested head, but you probably won't have a fever or other, flu-like symptoms. If you do, you probably have SARS. Just kidding!

THE FLU

If you don't have a cold, it's probably the flu. Estimates on the number of flu cases per year vary from 5% to 20% of the entire US population, though only estimates can be made as many people who contract the flu don't visit a doctor.

The flu is caused by a family of viruses called the orthomyxoviridae. All of the orthomyxoviridae are flu viruses, so you can imagine there are quite a few strains of the flu. More important to its infectivity, though, is two particular proteins it contains called Hemagglutinin Activity (HA) and Neuraminidase Activity (NA).

Before we get into the details of the surface proteins, let's discuss the basic structure of the influenza viruses. Orthomyxoviridae is a helical, enveloped virus, so while it can survive outside the body in respiratory droplets (those little drops that fly out when you sneeze or cough), once those dry up, the virus is no longer infectious. That's the good news. The bad news is that doesn't actually stop the virus from getting transmitted easily from person to person. The other relevant fact about the structure of the flu virus is that its genome is in eight segments, each one encoding for a particular protein. The HA and NA proteins each have their own gene segment, which is the critical factor in flu pandemics that sweep through, such as the Swine Flu in 2008 or the Spanish Flu in 1918. We'll talk about that in a bit, but hold on because it's fascinating.

We group the influenza viruses into three categories: A, B, and C. C causes only a mild illness in most people, so we rarely concern ourselves with that. A and B both cause the flu, with A being the worse of the two because it tends to change more and therefore be more infectious. Strains of influenza A viruses are also known to infect birds, pigs, horses, and seals, while B and C only infect humans. For the purposes of this book, we'll be discussing A and B strains.

The flu virus uses HA and NA to infect human cells. NA acts first by cleaving neuraminic acid, which is found in mucin. Mucin is the important component of mucus, which typically covers the cells in the human respiratory tract and protects the cells from damage and infection. By cutting up this acid, the mucin isn't able to perform its job and the HA can get to the cells.

HA is a protein that binds to sialic acid receptors on human cells, which are found on both red blood cells and the cells of the upper respiratory tract. Interestingly, the name hemagglutinin actually refers to the fact that viruses with HA on their surface cause aggregation (agglutination) of red blood cells (heme) when added to blood. When infecting people, though, the HA primarily targets the respiratory cells because we typically inhale the flu virus.

The act of HA binding to the sialic acid receptor triggers fusion of the viral membrane with the cell membrane, allowing the virus to dump its genetic material into the cell. Once inside, the virus does what viruses do and replicates, creating a bunch of copies and sending them out to infect other cells. Our immune system responds and creates the havoc we know as flu symptoms. Since we're all familiar with what the flu looks like, we won't discuss it here. Instead, let's look at why we get the flu a lot and why particular strains, like the Swine Flu, are so bad.

If you know a little about the immune system, you know that our body creates protective antibodies to prevent infection with the same virus or bacteria more than once. If our body can create antibodies to the HA receptor on a flu virus, we can actually prevent the virus from infecting our cells and we therefore have an immunity to that strain of the flu. Like colds, however, there are multiple strains, so we can get infected with different strains that have HA proteins different enough that our antibodies won't work. The true source of the flu viruses' potency, though, is antigenic drift and antigenic shift. We'll look at each of these in turn.

Antigenic drift is a fancy way of saying that the proteins made by the virus, also known as antigens, mutate slowly. In the infection section, I mentioned that RNA replication of viruses has no proofreading. Because of this, the wrong base will sometimes get added to the new strand of RNA. The base can have a positive, deleterious, or no effect. Because so many copies of the virus are made, even if half of the mutations are deleterious, one virus with a positive change can go on to make millions of copies and spread throughout the population.

Because antigenic drift takes place one mutation at a time,

the proteins that our antibodies recognize typically are unchanged enough that our antibodies can still recognize them. These slightly mutated strains often present in adults as upper respiratory infections similar to the common cold because healthy adults are able to fight off the virus quickly before it replicates and spreads throughout the body. The major problems occur when antigenic shift occurs.

Just by looking at the word shift, you can probably guess that it's worse than drift. After all, fishermen drift in their boats on a calm day. On the other hand, earthquakes cause the ground to shift. It's a much more dramatic change to the genetic material of the orthomyxovirus. Let's take a look at how it occurs.

The first thing you should know is that only strains of influenza A can undergo antigenic shift. The reason for this is, of course, the same thing that makes influenza A unique: there are strains of it that infect animals as well as humans. Normally, there's no crossover between the two in humans: the bird flu stays in birds, and the human flu stays in humans. However, pigs can get infected with both human and bird strains, as well as pig strains of the flu. Because of this, a pig cell can be infected with both a human and bird strain of the flu at the same time. Now, recall that the influenza genome is composed of eight separate segments of RNA. As each segment gets copied, it gets released into the cell, where it moves to the cell surface to be packaged into a new virus. With both a bird flu and human flu strains floating around, the wrong gene segment is packaged on occasion. If the gene segment happens to be for HA or NA, a major shift occurs. When a human virus gets repackaged with a bird (or pig, or horse, etc.) HA and NA, we call that antigenic shift. This is really bad news for us because that virus can infect humans, but our antibodies won't work on the new HA and NA because they're too different for our immune system to recognize. It's essentially like being infected with a totally new virus. This is where the global pandemics come from, since healthy adults have never been exposed to this viral strain and will get completely attacked by it before they can mount an immune response.

If you've ever wondered why these new viruses are called H1N1 and H5N1, the reason should be fairly clear now. The strains are given subtype numbers based on the new HA and NA that are packaged with the human virus, so H1N1 means that HA subtype 1 and NA subtype 1 were identified in this new strain. The good news for us is that many of these new viruses can't strongly infect humans—some can only be transmitted directly from the pigs or birds to humans, and some only have mild infectivity in humans. However, a highly infectious strain is possible, as we saw with the Spanish Flu in 1918. As a side note, this is the reason the pork industry is so highly regulated.

Since the flu has so many serotypes, it's hard to build a vaccine for it. That hasn't stopped us from trying, though. Each year, the vaccine manufacturers guess which three strains they think will be circulating through the population—usually two A strains and one B—and grow that virus into either a live attenuated or an inactivated vaccine. Some years they guess better than others, so having the vaccine won't necessarily stop you from getting the flu;

it just reduces your chances. And as far as treatment goes, there are a few antiviral options and more in the making, but right now, if you're a healthy adult, your best bet is to just wait it out.

HERPES, CHICKEN POX, AND THE KISSING DISEASE

When you hear the word herpes, you probably think STD. While one strain of herpes is an STD, that strain is just a small portion of all the herpes viruses that infect people each year. You may already know that cold sores are caused by a strain of herpes virus. Did you know, though, that the chickenpox virus is a member of the herpesviridae family? So is the virus that causes mononucleosis (the kissing disease). Over the next few pages, we'll discuss the herpes simplex virus, the Varicella-Zoster virus, and the Epstein-Barr virus. If you don't know which causes what just yet, you will soon.

Before we get into individual strains of herpes, let's take a look at the general characteristics of the herpesviridae family. All herpes viruses are enveloped viruses, and their genetic material is DNA. This is actually good news for us because DNA viruses have much more stable genomes and therefore are less likely to undergo mutations like the orthomyxoviridae and rhinoviruses do. Unlike many DNA viruses, though, herpes viruses all carry their own proteins for DNA synthesis. This is due, at least in part, to one of the unique factors of the herpes family, which is that they all can develop a latent state.

Latent infection can occur before or after the acute, apparent infection. While the virus lies latent, there is no sign of illness. Typically, latent infection is seen in nerve cells; we'll discuss this further when we talk about Varicella-Zoster Virus. During latent infection, the DNA does not get integrated into the infected cell, nor is the DNA replicated. Instead, only genes called Latent Associated Transcripts (LATs) are expressed during this time. The genes encode for a special type of RNA called microRNA, or miRNA for short (because biologists abbreviate everything). These miRNAs prevent the cell from responding to signals sent by the human body, telling the cell to die. Dying is bad news for the virus living inside the cell, so it keeps the cell alive in order to protect itself. This latent stage becomes important in the recurrence of certain diseases.

Another distinct part of herpes viruses is that they encode for a protein called thymidine kinase. Thymidine kinase is a DNA replication helper protein that converts one of the bases we discussed in the infection section to an active form of the nucleotide that can be used for DNA replication. This protein helps the virus replicate much more quickly than human DNA by providing it with the necessary bases, but it also works in our favor as a target for an antiviral. The antiviral acyclovir, which we briefly discussed earlier in this book, is nearly identical to the base (guanosine) that is converted by thymidine kinase, but instead of having a cyclical molecule on the side, it has a chain. When thymidine kinase converts acyclovir and it is used in place of guanosine in DNA replication, it halts the replication because more bases can't be added to the acyclovir. Acyclovir is a common treatment of herpes viruses.

Now that we understand the general aspects of the herpes virus, let's discuss specific diseases caused by these viruses. First up is the herpes simplex virus (HSV), of which there are two versions: HSV-1 and HSV-2. Don't confuse these with strains; there are many strains of both HSV-1 and HSV-2. These are just overarching categories.

HSV-1 is also known as oral herpes and is the most common cause of cold sores—about 90% of cold sores are caused by HSV-1. It's also incredibly common; about 90% of adults have had an HSV-1 infection at some point during their lives. This infection is often asymptomatic, due to the latent stage we discussed earlier. The virus gets into your body, often through the mouth, and breaks down the membranes between cells. This causes a giant cell, called a syncytium, to form, and your body's inflammatory response causes the area of infection to swell. This is what leads to the sores you see on your mouth, though they can be seen anywhere on the body.

After the initial infection, the virus travels up a nerve cell and lies dormant in the nerve cell body. During this period, it's nearly impossible for your body to find the virus, so it can't be wiped out. The virus lies in wait until it's triggered by something. Although scientists are still unsure all of the factors that can trigger the re-emergence of the virus, these factors do include sunlight, stress, and fever. The current theory is that stress turns on the viral replication cycle, and the virus travels down the nerve to the tissue. It's almost impossible to wipe out, either through antivirals or your immune system, because the virus can travel directly from cell to cell through the breakdown of cell membranes, rather than needing to travel through the bloodstream where the immune system can more easily attack. However, as you get older, recurrences become less frequent and may vanish altogether.

Cold sores themselves are fairly mild, but the HSV-1 virus can cause encephalitis, which is inflammation (usually caused by infection) of the brain. It occurs when the virus gets into the brain, rather than just lying dormant in the nerve cells. While it's an uncommon complication, when almost the entire population has HSV-1, it ends up being a significant percentage of all encephalitis cases. HSV-1 accounts for about 10% of encephalitis cases in the US, and it's fatal in 30-70% of cases. It is treatable with acyclovir, but many survivors of herpes encephalitis are left with permanent neurological damage. I wouldn't start panicking just yet, though. Encephalitis is still fairly rare.

The second form of herpes simplex, HSV-2, is commonly known as genital herpes. This form of herpes is usually, but not always, sexually transmitted. It can cause genital warts by the same mechanism that HSV-1 causes sores. These wars can be painful at first, but they do heal without scarring. While they often form on the genitals, they can form anywhere below the waist. The other bad news about HSV-2 is that it, too, is very hard to eliminate. Since it's often transmitted when there are no symptoms (since, let's be honest, genital warts are probably off-putting), you should know where your partner has been—or at least practice safe sex.

HSV-1 can occasionally cause genital herpes and HSV-2 can cause cold sores, so it isn't a hard and fast rule. Aside from the encephalitis, neither type will kill you, but they can be painful and embarrassing. Just remember that most of your friends and neighbors have herpes too.

The next virus in the herpes family, Varicella-Zoster, causes a disease most of us are intimately familiar with: chickenpox. The Varicella-Zoster Virus (VZV) has a structure similar to the other herpes viruses, but its DNA encodes for different envelope proteins that allow it to act differently from herpes simplex. The infection is primarily spread through respiratory secretions like coughing and sneezing and is highly contagious. Once the virus gets inside your system, it initially targets the respiratory tract, similar to a cold or the flu. However, VZV can also spread into the lymph system and therefore into your blood, a condition called viremia. You likely better know viremia, and its bacterial counterpart bacteremia, as sepsis. Septic shock, though, is pretty much just caused by bacteria. For viruses, the bloodstream is a common part of its infectivity and doesn't cause systemic shock.

When the virus spreads throughout the body, it causes the formation of syncytia, just like the herpes simplex virus. The resulting local areas of inflammation form small pustules that we know better as pox. The virus can be found in pustular (that is, pus-filled) lesions and can spread through touching the lesions, but if the lesion is crusted over, there's probably no virus inside. Overall infectivity of a patient starts about 2 days before the rash appears and lasts until the lesions are completely crusted.

Chickenpox itself isn't too bad, though it can lead to encephalitis, hepatitis (inflammation of the liver), and pneumonia in immunocompromised individuals. The more long-term issue that arises is that, like other herpes viruses, VZV is very good at lying dormant. Once your immune system has fought off the initial infection, a few of the viruses will retreat to your nerve cells near your spinal cord. Each vertebra in your spine has a nerve coming out each side; one to the right and one to the left. The nerve splits into multiple, smaller nerves that innervate organs, muscles, and skin in a particular area of the body. These areas typically cover the span of a few vertical inches and wrap from the spine around to the front center line of your body. When VZV retreats, it typically hides in just one of these nerves. There, it lies dormant, waiting for an opportunity to re-emerge. Since it isn't doing much of anything, your body isn't aware that it's even there, so the virus lives on.

Around the age of 50, your immunity to VZV begins to decline. The Varicella Zoster Virus sees the weakened defenses and seizes its opportunity to emerge. It spreads down the nerve to the particular area of skin innervated by that nerve. You initially feel pain, and a rash appears 3 days to 2 weeks later. The rash can be only one small spot or a few, but it typically is seen only on one side of the body in a lateral area because the nerve circles around half the body like a rope. This mild-appearing rash is incredibly painful to the touch, and this is what we call shingles. Shingles is the same virus as chickenpox, but it's the second infection when your body has some immunity to it and can control the virus when it emerges from its latent state. Interestingly, it took scientists some time to realize that chickenpox and shingles were caused by the same virus, since they appear so differently. This is the reason why VZV has two names: varicella was the name of chickenpox, while zoster referred to shingles before we realized they were the same virus.

A vaccine was approved for VZV in 1995 and was the subject of controversy, since many people debated the need and efficacy of the new vaccine. In studies, the vaccine was only effective on 70-90% of people, leaving 10-30% vulnerable to an infection as they got older. Additionally, people argued that chickenpox is a relatively mild disease and we shouldn't vaccinate against illnesses that are easily beaten and help boost our immune system. Nevertheless, the vaccine was approved based on the argument that VZV can lead to serious complications like encephalitis in a small subset of the population, and since it infects nearly everyone at one point or another, this can be a significant number of people.

Like herpes, acyclovir can be used to treat VZV, though it's primarily used for shingles and varicella encephalitis, not ordinary chickenpox.

The last type of herpes virus we'll discuss is called Epstein-Barr Virus (EBV), but it's better known as mononucleosis, mono, or the kissing disease. Mono is interesting in that it is primarily a disease only in developed countries because EBV is asymptomatic in children. Since underdeveloped countries tend to have less hygienic practices, viruses spread quickly and most people have been infected by EBV before they reach puberty. This infection grants them immunity to reinfections, and they therefore never develop mononucleosis.

In developed countries, EBV is less common, but that means that people tend to get the infection at a later age. The virus spreads through saliva, which is where the nickname "the kissing disease" comes from. It also explains why it's very common at universities, where there's a lot of kissing and drink-sharing going on. When the virus is transmitted, it initially infects the cells in the nose and throat, where it replicates and is released. The virus then spreads into the bloodstream, where it targets a particular type of immune cell: the B cell we discussed earlier.

Once inside the B cells, the viruses not only replicate, but they also activate a lot of the B cells they infect. Activating a B cell means that it starts producing antibodies to the particular pathogen it's designed to attack. In the case of mono, the B cell gets improperly activated, so it might target a cell in your body rather than the invader it's designed to attack.

Luckily for us, the B cells aren't a critical part of fighting off the EBV. Instead, T cells provide the cell-mediated immunity needed to kill off the cells hosting the virus and eliminate it from your body.

EBV has an incubation period of about 4-6 weeks. The symptoms then begin with the typical fatigue and muscle ache that accompanies nearly every virus. After a week or two, a fever, sore throat, and swollen lymph nodes appear. What is distinctive about EBV is that the fever can last over a month. After a few weeks, the swollen lymph nodes progress to an enlarged spleen. This happens because the spleen is a part of the immune system, as are lymph nodes, and the proliferation of active B cells and T cells causes an increase in the cells and fluid in the lymph system. This then leads to more cells in the spleen, which causes it to enlarge.

Most people eventually fight the virus off, with symptoms lasting 2-4 weeks. However, the tiredness and difficulty concentrating can last for months after the other symptoms dissipate. Like other herpes viruses, the illness rarely results in death, but it can lead to encephalitis and other complications of the central nervous system that lead to death. This is pretty rare, though. There is one serious long-term complication, however. Infection with EBV has been associated with a type of cancer called Burkitt's lymphoma, which is a cancer of B cells. There's a strong link in Africa, with 90% of the cases of Burkitt's lymphoma associated with a previous EBV infection. In the US, the link is less strong (15% of Burkitt's lymphoma patients have EBV antibodies showing they had a prior infection), but both Hodgkin's and non-Hodgkin's lymphomas have also been associated with EBV.

MEASLES, MUMPS, AND RUBELLA

Because measles, mumps, and rubella all come in the same vaccine, I've lumped them together in this book. However, while measles and mumps are caused by the same family of viruses, rubella comes from a different family altogether. We'll discuss the differences as we look at each disease, but I wanted to set the record straight before we all get confused.

Measles and mumps are both members of the paramyxoviridae family. Those of you who have been paying close attention will notice the similarities between the name of this family and that of the influenza family (orthomyxoviridae). There are a number of similarities between the two families. Both are enveloped with a helical structure and negative-strand RNA. The one difference in their makeup (aside from the obvious differences in RNA sequence) is that paramyxoviridae have one continuous RNA strand, while orthomyxoviridae have a genome composed of eight separate segments. This is a bit of a relief for us, since it means we don't have to worry about antigenic shift for paramyxoviridae.

The paramyxoviridae family contains measles, mumps, respiratory syncytial virus (RSV), and parainfluenza, the last of which you can probably guess resembles influenza. We're only going to discuss measles and mumps in this section.

Like the flu viruses, the envelope of the paramyxoviridae contains HA and NA, which allow the viruses to get through mucus and attach to cells in the respiratory tract. One additional protein separates the para- and orthomyxoviridae, though: the fusion protein. As you might guess, the fusion protein causes fusion, specifically of the cell membranes. This protein is used to form giant cells, or syncytia, which we discussed in the herpes section.

Measles is caused by a specific virus in the paramyxoviridae family called the morbillivirus. Measles is highly infectious and is transmitted via respiratory droplets from coughing and sneezing, so it spreads easily and in a manner similar to the flu. There's only one strain of morbillivirus. Because of this and its infectivity, it was primarily seen in children before the advent of the MMR vaccine. Now it isn't seen in many people at all.

Once inside a person, morbillivirus use HA to attach to cells and release its genetic material into the cell. As the virus starts replicating, there's no rash but the patient is infectious. People in this stage typically develop a fever and have runny noses, a cough, inflammation of the membrane covering the eye called the conjunctiva, and they dislike light. Meanwhile, the virus is replicating and being released inside the body, and eventually it spreads into the bloodstream. As the virus begins to infect the cells that line the inside of blood vessel, T cells specific for morbillivirus get activated and attack the cells that are infected with the virus.

Since the cells lining the blood vessels are infected, some of these cells die under the attack, allowing blood to leak out. This leakage in the capillaries of the skin is what causes the characteristic rash of measles to appear. Because the initial infection is in the upper airways, the rash starts at the head of the patient and spreads down toward the feet. It then disappears in the same pattern, with the head clearing up first and the feet last.

A day or two before the rash appears, characteristic Koplik's spots appear in the inside the mouth on the cheeks. These spots are red with small blue-white spots in the center. If you see these inside your mouth, you can be fairly sure you have measles.

Like so many of the other viruses we've discussed, measles is unlikely to kill you, but there is the potential of encephalitis, which is fatal in about 10% of the encephalitis cases.

Mumps is caused by the cleverly-named mumps virus, and it spreads the same way as measles. It, just like measles, infects the cells of the respiratory tract. The virus is asymptomatic for up to 21 days, after which you develop a fever, feel tired, and have no appetite. Unlike measles, mumps doesn't cause a rash. Instead, it targets glands inside your body called the parotid glands. These glands are salivary glands found near the mouth, and when the virus gets inside the glands, they swell. This causes the side of the patient's face to swell. It's generally very painful. The next step for the virus is to head down to the testes in males, which swell as well. If both testes are infected and swell, this can cause sterility due to the pressure on the testes. Sterility only occurs if the patient is past puberty, though. Eventually, your body will clear out the infection.

Now we come to rubella. As I mentioned, rubella is not a paramyxovirus, so it functions differently. Rubella is caused by the rubivirus, which is a member of the togaviridae family. Rubella is also known as German measles because of its resemblance to measles. Rubella is also spread through respiratory droplets and initially appears as a flu-like illness. After a few days, a rash appears on the forehead that spreads down the limbs and torso. You can see the resemblance to measles here. However, the rash only lasts for three days and cannot cause encephalitis, so it acts a lot like a mild version of measles. The big problem with rubella, and the reason it is vaccinated against, is that it can cross the placental barrier in pregnant women and cause severe congenital defects. If the virus occurs early in the pregnancy, it can cause cataracts, mental retardation, and deafness, among other defects. If the mother has either had rubella prior to pregnancy or has had the vaccine, there's nothing to worry about. The issues only occur when a non-vaccinated pregnant woman gets infected with rubella for the first time.

Speaking of vaccines, did you know there's a vaccine for MMR? I hope so, I mentioned it about twenty times. The vaccine is the only defense we have against measles, mumps, and rubella (aside from our own natural defenses, of course). The vaccine is a mix of the three viruses (morbillivirus, mumps virus, and rubivirus) and it is a live attenuated vaccine. As we know, this means that no adjuvant is needed and our body develops antibodies to the viruses just like a real infection. What it also means, though, is that the vaccine can't be given to pregnant women because it would act the same as an infection with the actual rubivirus and cross the placental barrier. Women should all have this vaccine before having children.

HIV

Now that we've covered the more common viruses, let's talk about the rarer and scarier ones. Arguably the scariest virus in existence, Human Immunodeficiency Virus (HIV) only entered the human population in late 1980/early 1981. Despite this, it's the most researched virus in the world, and anyone who knows even a little about HIV can guess why. Because of all this research, HIV is one of the best-understood viruses, which gives us options to fight its replication. While we can hold the virus at bay, HIV is not curable (with few notable exceptions).

As I mentioned earlier, HIV is a retrovirus, so it transcribes its RNA to DNA using an RNA-dependent DNA polymerase. HIV is not the only retrovirus, but it is certainly the best known and studied. Other retroviruses include oncoviruses, which cause cancers and other neurologic disorders, and endogenous viruses, which are retroviral sequences that have been permanently integrated into the genome of the host cell. This isn't really an issue because they aren't doing anything, but it's a concern with the possibility of transplantation from animals, such as pigs, into humans. There's a concern that these endogenous sequences will be activated when they get transplanted into a human.

HIV is a member of the lentivirus genus, which includes retroviruses that have a slow onset of disease and whose primary targets are neurologic cells and the immune system.

HIV is an enveloped virus that must be transmitted either sexually or through blood transfusions. Luckily for us, it isn't that infectious, since it can only attach to a receptor on T cells, rather than a common cell surface receptor like colds and the flu do. Inside the capsid of the HIV virus, it carries 2 copies of its positive-strand RNA genome, along with three critical proteins called reverse transcriptase (RT), integrase (IN), and protease (PT). Its envelope contains two proteins, TM and SU, which it uses to attach to human T cells.

When the HIV virus gets into the human body, it aims for those T cells as if its life depends on it—which it does. T cells circulate throughout the blood, looking for invaders, so this works well for HIV. It is an invader, after all. When HIV finds a T cell, the SU protein on its surface attaches to a receptor on the T cell called CD4. Without going into too many details on the immune system, all you should know is that the CD4 receptor is used by T cells to help get the immune system going. This receptor is only found on a subset of T cells, so there's only a small percentage of cells that HIV can target. Once SU is bound, TM is used to fuse cell membranes, turning them into a giant syncytia where the virus can take advantage of the DNA replication machinery of multiple cells. It's a pretty clever system for the virus, but it's a bad system for us. In case there weren't enough random letters floating around, SU and TM both have alternate names: gp120 and gp41, respectively.

Once inside the cell, reverse transcriptase is used to reverse transcribe the RNA to DNA. This is its RNA-dependent DNA polymerase, and it's a major target for HIV drugs (commonly called anti-retrovirals, which you can now understand). Integrase is then used to integrate the newly-transcribed viral DNA into the host cell. The viral DNA is transcribed back to RNA using our cell's machinery, and then the RNA is translated into a number of proteins. Three of these proteins have a well-understood function: GAG, POL, and ENV.

At this point, protease shows up. A protease is a simply a protein that cleaves other proteins. The protease in HIV cuts the three proteins that were translated into smaller proteins that can be used to form new HIV viruses. GAG is cut into smaller proteins that make up the capsid of the virus. POL is chopped into new copies of RT, IN, and PT. ENV is cleaved into SU and TM.

There are a number of other proteins found in HIV, but they aren't critical to understanding how HIV functions.

HIV is clever because by targeting a specific cell in your immune system, it weakens your body's ability to fight off invaders. This works out really well for the virus because it sits in the cell, making copies of itself and sending them out to infect other T cells. Over time, your bone marrow, which produces the cells of your immune system, can't keep up with the demand for new T cells, and the total number in your body drops. As the level drops, your body's ability to fight off infection drops as well. Normal T cell levels are 1000 cells per microliter of blood. A person with HIV will have a slowly decreasing number, and when the number of cells drops below 200 per microliter, we say the patient has AIDS.

Remember in all the other sections when I mentioned that immunocompromised people were at risk for all sorts of complications? People with AIDS are a classic example of those immunocompromised people. A virus, bacteria, or fungus that to you and me would be easy to fight can be lethal in an HIV-infected person, since they lack the necessary T cells to rid their body of that pathogen. HIV, by itself, won't kill a person. However, without an immune system, some other pathogen will.

You may be wondering now why we don't develop a vaccine to get rid of HIV. The problem lies in the ability of the HIV virus to mutate, particularly in critical areas like the gene that codes for SU. The mutations in HIV occur at a very high rate, even for an RNA virus, and they occur in a way so as to preserve the function of the virus. Like I said, it's a very clever virus. Because of the high mutation rate, there are a lot of versions of HIV, and they're constantly changing so that any vaccine we develop will be almost instantly obsolete.

As far as treatment goes, all current medications are focused on stopping the replication of HIV and the spread of resistant viruses. There are drugs that target RT and there are drugs that target PT. The way in which most HIV-positive patients are treated is with a combination of drugs, called HAART, which means Highly Active AntiRetroviral Therapy. The concept is to use multiple drugs with different mechanisms of action in order to limit viral replication even if the virus mutates and one of the drugs becomes ineffective. The particular combination depends on the patient and the virus and involves some trial and error in order to find a combination that is both effective and tolerable for the patient. New drugs are constantly being tested, and the virus is constantly mutating to avoid these drugs. All in all, I'd highly recommend avoiding the virus.

HEMORRHAGIC FEVERS

No book written in 2014 would be complete without a discussion of Ebola. It's just one of many, many viruses out there, some of which are far worse than Ebola, but we'll talk about it anyway. After all, it's interesting if nothing else. Ebola is a hemorrhagic fever, which means that it causes you to bleed. Hemorrhage is just a fancy word for bleeding. They occur when viruses infect the lining of blood vessels, causing the vessels to become leaky and allow blood out into your body cavities and space beneath the skin. On top of this, your immune system turns against the cells that are infected, killing them off and further damaging the integrity of the blood vessels.

When too much blood leaves the vessels, your body becomes hypotensive, which is the opposite of hypertension and is also a very bad thing. Without enough blood in the vessels, you don't get enough oxygen to your organs, leading to organ failure. If left untreated, organs and other under-oxygenated parts of your body begin to die. Eventually, you die as well.

Of course, hospitals can treat hypovolemic shock by giving more fluids and blood intravenously, and eventually your body will kill the virus and you'll recover. Hemorrhagic fevers aren't necessarily going to kill you, but they certainly can. Let's take a look at the viruses that cause these fevers.

Hemorrhagic fevers can be caused by a number of viruses from various families. The first family we'll discuss today, the flaviviridae, causes two diseases you may be more familiar with than Ebola: dengue fever and yellow fever. Both of these viruses are transmitted from human to human by mosquitos, specifically the *Aedes aegypti* mosquito (in case that ever comes up in trivia). It's rare that they actually cause hemorrhagic fever, so we won't discuss the mechanistic details. Typically, dengue begins 2-7 days after the virus is transmitted to the patient via mosquito bite. It starts with a high fever, headache, back pain, and severe muscle pain that gives rise to its colloquial name, break bone fever. The fever comes and goes for 4-6 days, after which point most people recover. In a small percentage of cases (about 0.25%), the disease progresses to hemorrhagic fever. It occurs via the mechanism we discussed earlier, where the virus gets into the blood vessels and damages the cells. The not-so-great part about that small percentage is that there are an estimated 100 million cases of dengue fever worldwide each year, so 0.25% still means that about 250,000 cases of dengue progress to hemorrhagic fever.

Yellow fever is very similar to dengue, with a few differences. First, monkeys are the host for the disease, so you need to be bitten by a mosquito that first bit an infected monkey in order to get the disease. This means that there are far fewer cases of yellow fever than dengue each year: only about 200,000. On the flip side, about 15% of the cases of yellow fever progress to hemorrhagic fever, so patients who have yellow fever are much more likely to get hemorrhagic fever. About 20% of these patients with hemorrhagic fever will die.

In severe cases of yellow fever, the liver, kidney, and heart get involved. The liver stops functioning properly, leading to a build-up of bilirubin in the bloodstream, since the liver normally clears this biomolecule. Excess bilirubin causes jaundice, which makes the patients appear yellow. Hence, the name yellow fever.

Luckily, there is a vaccine for yellow fever, and if you're traveling between certain countries, you might be asked to show proof that you've had the vaccine. It comes in two forms, oral and injected, and I can tell you from personal experience that the oral vaccine causes stomach aches. Still, I'll take some mild stomach problems over turning yellow and possibly dying.

The bunyaviridae family is responsible for a number of hemorrhagic fevers, including Crimean-Congo hemorrhagic fever, Rift Valley hemorrhagic fever, and Hantavirus. Crimean-Congo and Rift Valley are both spread by arthropods, which means ticks, sandflies, and mosquitos. Both have animal hosts—sheep and cattle, among others—and both are pretty rare, so we aren't going to discuss them in detail. Just know that they exist and can cause hemorrhagic fevers.

Hantavirus is a bit different from other members of the bunyaviridae family in that it is transmitted by rodents, rather than arthropods. There are two types of hantavirus: Hantaan virus, which causes Korean hemorrhagic fever, and Sin Nombre virus, which causes Hantavirus Pulmonary Syndrome.

Can you guess where Hantaan virus is seen? If you guessed Korea, China, and Russia, you guessed right! The virus was seen in UN troops during the Korean War, and in 1976 it was isolated from a rodent in Korea, hence the name. The severe form of Korean hemorrhagic fever is called Hemorrhagic Fever with Renal Syndrome (HFRS). People get infected with the virus by inhaling aerosols of rodent output, meaning urine, feces, and saliva. In an acute infection, the virus gets into the kidney and causes nephritis (inflammation of the kidney) that leads to insufficient renal function and can eventually lead to renal failure. The kidneys are pretty important in clearing unwanted substances from the blood, not to mention producing urine, so not having functioning kidneys is an issue. On top of this, hemorrhage can occur, leading to hypovolemic shock. If this happens, it's fatal in 5-15% of cases.

Sin Nombre virus was first recognized in 1993 with an outbreak of a severe respiratory illness in the southwestern US. People eventually figured out that deer mice were hosting a new strain of hantavirus, which for some odd reason they decided to name Sin Nombre ('without name' in Spanish). Sin Nombre doesn't actually cause hemorrhagic fevers, unlike most other bunyaviridae, but it does lead to pulmonary edema, which is when the lungs fill with fluid. Sin Nombre doesn't appear to currently transmit person to person, but it has a fatality rate of over 30%.

There are a number of other viruses that cause hemorrhagic fevers, but most are relatively rare. So to wrap things up, let's talk about Ebola.

Ebola is caused by the Ebola virus and is a member of the

Filoviridae family. Filoviruses are enveloped RNA viruses that look like long threads, and there are only two known types: Marburg and Ebola. Marburg virus is named for the city in Germany in which it was first discovered. It was seen in 1967 in lab techs who interacted with tissues of African green monkeys that were imported into the city. This disease appears to be rare, though there have been a few recorded cases of it in various countries in Africa.

Ebola, on the other hand, seems to occur in sporadic outbreaks and was first noted in 1976. Cases of severe hemorrhagic fevers were seen in Sudan and the Congo (known at the time as Zaire). The total number of infected persons has been historically low, with only 1850 cases recorded between 1976 and 2004. Unfortunately, 1200 of those infected people died, giving Ebola the highest mortality rate of all the hemorrhagic fevers. Part of this high mortality rate could be due to the fact that the outbreaks occur in remote areas of Africa without much access to healthcare, so the patients don't receive the supportive treatment they need to survive the infection. Estimates of the death rate of Marburg and Ebola are between 25 and 90%, depending on the strand that is circulating that year.

The Ebola virus is spread through contact with bodily fluids from an infected person, and while it's speculated that there is an animal host for the virus, it has yet to be discovered.

Once the virus is inside the patient, it takes about 4-10 days for enough viruses to accumulate and cause symptoms. It can infect a wide variety of cells in the body, so it isn't restricted by its need to hunt down a specific type of cell. It typically replicates inside two and a half types of cells, called monocytes, macrophages, and dendritic cells, which are all part of your body's initial immune response to infection. This gives the virus an immunosuppressive effect, making it harder to fight off infections. I say two and a half because monocytes and macrophages are basically the same cell located in different parts of your body. The virus then spreads through the lymph system and blood to the liver and spleen.

The first symptoms are, like so many other viruses, flu-like. This makes it pretty hard to diagnose Ebola in early stages of the disease. A number of other symptoms can occur, such as nausea, vomiting, chest pain, cough, headache, confusion, and even comas. After about a week, a rash appears.

As the disease progresses and infects the liver, the liver stops synthesizing enough of the proteins needed for coagulation, which may be part of the cause of the hemorrhage. Despite this, the hemorrhage itself is only present in about half of affected patients and massive blood loss is uncommon.

Because of the rarity of Ebola, there's no standard treatment and no vaccine. Current treatment primarily involves treating the symptoms and providing supportive care, like blood transfusions and IV nutrition. There are some antivirals and vaccines in development, but for the time being, the strategy is to quarantine and wait it out.

FINAL THOUGHTS

Viruses are one of the biggest problems health care workers face today, and by extension, all of us. Viruses can spread quickly, mutate even faster, and are hard to eliminate. There are vast numbers of them, and new ones arise more frequently than anyone would like. They cause diseases, yes, but they also can cause long-term consequences like cancer.

So what can we do? For now, keep learning. We don't fully understand viruses or how they work, so we can't fully understand how to stop them. In the future, we'll probably learn that half the things we thought were true in this book are wrong. Keep learning, and if you're interested in more science, don't forget to check out the other *Layman's Guide to Medical School* books. Until next time!

ABOUT THE AUTHOR

COLLEEN FLESHMAN is a first-year medical student who has always been fascinated with the human body. She finds textbooks annoying for the dry way in which they approach interesting subjects and always wished someone would publish versions of her textbooks that were written by humans, rather than science robots. She currently lives in Florida.

SOURCES

Acosta EP, Flexner C. Chapter 58. Antiviral Agents (Nonretroviral). In: Brunton LL, Chabner BA, Knollmann BC. eds. Goodman & Gilman's The Pharmacological Basis of Therapeutics, 12e. New York, NY: McGraw-Hill; 2011.http://accessmedicine.mhmedical.com.ezproxy.fau.edu/content.aspx?bookid=374&Sectionid=41266269. Accessed December 22, 2014.

Brooks GF, Carroll KC, Butel JS, Morse SA, Mietzner TA. Chapter 38. Arthropod-Borne and Rodent-Borne Viral Diseases. In: Brooks GF, Carroll KC, Butel JS, Morse SA, Mietzner TA. eds. Jawetz, Melnick, & Adelberg's Medical Microbiology, 26e. New York, NY: McGraw-Hill; 2013.http://accessmedicine.mhmedical.com.ezproxy.fau.edu/content.aspx?bookid=504&Sectionid=40999960. Accessed November 21, 2014.

Brooks GF, Carroll KC, Butel JS, Morse SA, Mietzner TA. Chapter 29. General Properties of Viruses. In: Brooks GF, Carroll KC, Butel JS, Morse SA, Mietzner TA. eds. Jawetz, Melnick, & Adelberg's Medical Microbiology, 26e.New York, NY: McGraw-Hill; 2013.http://accessmedicine.mhmedical.com.ezproxy.fau.edu/content.aspx?bookid=504&Sectionid=40999951. Accessed November 28, 2014.

Brooks GF, Carroll KC, Butel JS, Morse SA, Mietzner TA. Chapter 39. Orthomyxoviruses (Influenza Viruses). In: Brooks GF, Carroll KC, Butel JS, Morse SA, Mietzner TA. eds. Jawetz, Melnick, & Adelberg's Medical Microbiology, 26e. New York, NY: McGraw-Hill; 2013.http://accessmedicine.mhmedical.com.ezproxy.fau.edu/conte

nt.aspx?bookid=504&Sectionid=40999961. Accessed December 27, 2014.

Cohen JI. Chapter 181. Epstein-Barr Virus Infections, Including Infectious Mononucleosis. In: Longo DL, Fauci AS, Kasper DL, Hauser SL, Jameson J, Loscalzo J. eds. Harrison's Principles of Internal Medicine, 18e. New York, NY: McGraw-Hill; 2012.http://accessmedicine.mhmedical.com.ezproxy.fau.edu/conte nt.aspx?bookid=331&Sectionid=40726937. Accessed December 31, 2014.

Dolin R. Chapter 186. Common Viral Respiratory Infections. In: Longo DL, Fauci AS, Kasper DL, Hauser SL, Jameson J, Loscalzo J. eds. Harrison's Principles of Internal Medicine, 18e. New York, NY: McGraw-Hill; 2012.http://accessmedicine.mhmedical.com.ezproxy.fau.edu/conte nt.aspx?bookid=331&Sectionid=40726943. Accessed November 16, 2014.

Levinson W. Chapter 39. RNA-Enveloped Viruses. In: Levinson W. eds. Review of Medical Microbiology & Immunology, 12e. New York, NY: McGraw-Hill; 2012.http://accessmedicine.mhmedical.com.ezproxy.fau.edu/conte nt.aspx?bookid=400&Sectionid=42098503. Accessed November 16, 2014.

Raasch RH. Chapter 158. Pharmacology of Antimicrobics, Antifungals, and Antivirals. In: Tintinalli JE, Stapczynski J, Ma O, Cline DM, Cydulka RK, Meckler GD, T. eds. Tintinalli's Emergency Medicine: A Comprehensive Study Guide, 7e.New York, NY: McGraw-Hill; 2011.http://accessmedicine.mhmedical.com.ezproxy.fau.edu/conte nt.aspx?bookid=348&Sectionid=40381635. Accessed December 22, 2014.

Ropper AH, Samuels MA, Klein JP. Chapter 33. Viral Infections of the Nervous System, Chronic Meningitis, and Prion Diseases. In: Ropper AH, Samuels MA, Klein JP. eds. Adams & Victor's Principles of Neurology, 10e. New York, NY: McGraw-Hill; 2014.http://accessmedicine.mhmedical.com.ezproxy.fau.edu/conte

nt.aspx?bookid=690&Sectionid=50910884. Accessed December 29, 2014.

Ryan KJ, Ray C. Enteroviruses. In: Ryan KJ, Ray C. eds. Sherris Medical Microbiology, Sixth Edition. New York, NY: McGraw-Hill; 2014.http://accessmedicine.mhmedical.com.ezproxy.fau.edu/content.aspx?bookid=1020&Sectionid=56968712. Accessed November 21, 2014.

Ryan KJ, Ray C. Chapter 14. Herpesviruses. In: Ryan KJ, Ray C. eds. Sherris Medical Microbiology, 5e. New York, NY: McGraw-Hill; 2010.http://accessmedicine.mhmedical.com.ezproxy.fau.edu/content.aspx?bookid=375&Sectionid=40299141. Accessed November 17, 2014.

Schuchat A, Jackson LA. Chapter 122. Immunization Principles and Vaccine Use. In: Longo DL, Fauci AS, Kasper DL, Hauser SL, Jameson J, Loscalzo J.eds. Harrison's Principles of Internal Medicine, 18e. New York, NY: McGraw-Hill; 2012. http://accessmedicine.mhmedical.com.ezproxy.fau.edu/content.aspx?bookid=331&Sectionid=40726864. Accessed December 22, 2014.